The
POSSIBILITY
of BALANCE

The
POSSIBILITY
of BALANCE

NAMRATAA ARORA SINGH

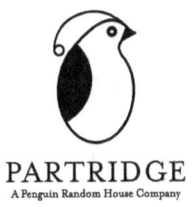

PARTRIDGE
A Penguin Random House Company

To order additional copies of this book, contact
Partridge India
000 800 10062 62
orders.india@partridgepublishing.com

www.partridgepublishing.com/india

PRAISE FOR THE POSSIBILITY OF BALANCE

"The Possibility of Balance is a guidebook for women, specifically mothers who want to consider making their dreams come true. Through this book, Namrataa invites you to imagine what life could be like if... to leap beyond your considerations, excuses, and reasons that you cannot have your life be the way you want and start going for your dreams. If you find yourself wanting more in your current life, then read this handbook for living a fulfilled and balanced life."

Cherie Carter-Scott, Ph.D. MCC
author of
If Life is a Game, These are the Rules
and
The Gift of Motherhood

The acid test of the usefulness of a self-help book is whether or not the reader can actually implement the guidance it delivers. Namrataa has ensured that her pearls of wisdom are not only absolutely on-target but are easily able to be implemented. Test passed!

And why would you listen to Namrataa? Simply because she has been in the same place and situation as you! She has personal, real-life experience and has faced, and overcome, the same challenges as her readers are facing. She knows what needs to be done - and delivers the answers in this easy-to-read book.

Read her insights, follow her guidance and your life will be all the more satisfying as a result!

Lynne Elder DipM MCIM CPC,
Founder and Principal of SheSmart Marketing

CONTENTS

To my favourite women:

My daughter, *Siddhangana*, who is the
reason that I started my journey of
self-discovery and balance

and

My mother, *Shashi*, who has never given
up her pursuit for balance in all spheres of her
life and continues to be my inspiration

ACKNOWLEDGEMENT

I am grateful to the following people for their contribution to this book:

- The participants of my signature program 'My Life, By Design', whose progress in accomplishing their chosen goals has been my inspiration through this journey,
- Aruna Lakshmanan, for being the person to pull together all my writing, content mining, and research,
- Asawari Salwan, for introducing me to Aruna and for being my co-passenger in my writing journey,
- My family, for their never-ending support and encouragement,
- Justin Rabindra Photography for my picture

HOW TO READ THIS BOOK

You could, of course, take the usual format of reading this book—that is, end to end—but I am not sure how useful this book might be for you.

This is meant to be a *life guide* for women. What would work best is for you to pick a theme, an area of your life that you are currently struggling with, and read the chapters related to that theme. Sleep over it. The way I found self-help books to be most useful to me was when I read a specific section at a particular point of time in my life. Some books, I must admit, I have read over and over till I have interpreted them in different ways at different junctures in my life journey.

Coaches usually recommend writing a journal when one is planning on making a big change in one's life. I would recommend writing for everyone. Pick your format, frequency and whatever else you need to. Writing, I find, is the best way of self-reflection. It is uncluttered with the thoughts of others around us, and it is our purest form of expression. Writing your thoughts while you read this book would help you take action.

DO YOU LIVE BY DESIGN?

When was the last time you thought about a different kind of life?

Have you ever had a moment in which you started to question why you are doing what you are doing and wondered what a different life would be like?

The good news is that a different life is possible. The bad news is that not many of us recognise this fact. Think about it. For big decisions we make at work, we have a goal and we have a plan to get to that goal. When it comes to our personal lives, we get caught up in living life one day at a time.

What would happen if we were to document our dreams? What if we were to treat our dreams as goals and had a plan to get to those goals? Could it be true that we fear success more than we fear failure? That might explain why, perhaps, we believe our dreams are best left unwritten and unmentioned to those around us. Sadly, sometimes, even to ourselves.

What if your dreams became real? Are you ready to live them?

If yes, start with a blank sheet of paper. Draw up your dreams. Depict your life as you would like it to be on a typical day. Start with what you might want to do in the morning. What kind of work do you engage in through the day? What does your home look like? Where would you be living? Who are the people you want to be around? What really helps is to chart out a week in as much detail as possible. In an ideal life, what would a typical week look like?

This, superimposed with your priorities and your passion, can throw up some interesting revelations, often resulting in stark and revealing conclusions. For instance, you may realise that you are really not in the right profession as that does not play to your strengths or that you may, really, be in the right profession but need to fundamentally restructure your work life in a way that it fits into the ideal week much better. Perhaps even consider relocating to a different city.

Now, think about *what is stopping you from making this a reality.* Are these real obstacles?

Being purposeful about whatever we do is the ultimate way of life.

Do you believe you are ready to challenge yourself and step out of your comfort zone to create a better life?

If you are convinced that a different life is what you want to focus on creating, the rest of this book will guide you with simple and practical tips that have helped moms across the globe. Some chapters in this book might not appeal to you, and some might not even be relevant, but I do urge you to evaluate them and to celebrate each and every change you are able to make in your life.

Section 1

ME

WHAT IS THE VALUE OF YOUR TIME?

How do you start your day? Do you get up in a rush, wondering what to cook or scamper to get your child ready for school? We often fall prey to the clock, and before we know it, the morning has morphed into the rest of the day, and we have been consumed by events and people around us. The result is our favourite quote: 'I don't have time!' How can we possibly make time for ourselves when the first thought after we have woken up is about getting our long list of tasks done before the day ends?

Rise with the sun, preferably a bit before it does! An often-quoted formula for success by some of the world's most popular leaders is an early start to the day. That does not mean getting up and then hanging around, waiting for the panic of the day's routine to take over your life. It simply means that we start the day with a focus on ourselves.

How can we make our start of the day about a healthier version of us? Some of us start with yoga or simply a morning walk while others have adopted a meditation or fitness regime. Many moms who have participated in my one-day workshop on life design have spoken about the impossibility of making this happen owing to the lack of support at home.

After two months of the workshop, during follow-up sessions, women have shared the following ways they achieved consistency in their practice. Some found a friend who knocked on their door when it was time for a walk, some started to take their baby out with them so they were not worried while they were out, and some even considered altering the time of their domestic helpers (perhaps more relevant for Asian countries). Moms who have determined they were going to make things work have, indeed, reported success in accomplishing many goals.

My challenge to you is to bring forth your best problem-solving abilities as you probably might do at your workplace. We all know this: if we want something bad enough, we will find a way to make it happen.

This is not just about getting up early. It is about a purposeful, positive start to a day. It is about being conscious of our choices right from the moment we get up.

Having discussed about designing your life the way you would like it to be and starting your day early, let us now think about adding a price tag to your time. For many of us, our price tag is what others assign to us. The salary we make or the brand of clothes we think we should buy from the shops we think we should visit, define our worth. While that does not mean that we start splurging the money we do not really have, it certainly does mean that each of us could do with a fresh look at who we want to be perceived as. The key question to ask is, *what is my time worth?*

If we peg the value of our time at a premium, why would we want to spend time waiting in a queue to buy groceries when we can get someone else to do that for us? If we believe we are ready for the next promotion, why would we settle for a lower salary and give up negotiating after a point? If we believe we are capable of doing much greater things, why do we not start doing them?

Reflection

- *What one change would you want to make in your life in the next one month?*

- *How do you plan on making it happen?*

HOW MUCH TIME DO YOU SPEND ON YOURSELF?

A very important aspect of being independent is emotional freedom. Some of us already have a set of friends that we hang out with and are able to have fun without our families around. Too often, those of us with families, especially those of us with children, tend to start believing that there is no happiness for us outside of our family. We tend to make excuses when our friends ask us out for a movie or if we need to travel without our family. While the emotional attachment is good and understandable, this could pose a risk over time. Not being able to find ways to be happy outside of your family might leave you with no ways of being happy when children grow up and move out for further studies or when your spouse travels for long periods.

Finding your own space, developing your own interests and hobbies, having your own ways of having fun do not make you a selfish person or mean that you do not love your family. These, in fact, go a long way in ensuring your long-term happiness and, as a result, the happiness of those around you, including, of course, your loved ones.

It is healthy to do things and to have your own life. That is, in fact, the very essence of true independence. When was the last time you took off by yourself and let yourself soak in a place?

With the plethora of women travel clubs appearing on Facebook and other media, more and more women are finding solace in the fact that they would now be able to travel in groups.

For many women, especially mothers, leisure travel, surprisingly, is often considered a chore—when travelling with kids, that is. It might be the fact that most times it is the woman who is behind planning a vacation and, more importantly, packing for it too. It might also be that there is an unstated expectation that once back, the woman would, somehow, get the house back in order and the house would start functioning immediately.

It is, however, possible to turn a rather exhausting travel into a thrilling adventure.

To begin with, consider planning a solo travel to a place where you might know someone but have never visited. Travelling to an unknown place with nobody that one knows can be a bit stressful, and the idea is really to de-stress and have fun.

Travelling on work could be made fun if it were extended by a day here and there, but it could become more stressful to manage the logistics. Hence, planning a separate travel is perhaps much better. Just take off!

Reflection

- *What activities do you engage in when you have the most fun by yourself?*

HOW IMPORTANT IS YOUR HEALTH?

Physical fitness is not only one of the most important keys to a healthy body, it is the basis of a dynamic and creative intellectual activity.

—John F. Kennedy

Many moms I spoke with expressed health and fitness as their primary concern. Some admitted that they are unable to follow a routine due to "lack of time" (the world's most famous excuse!) while others shared tips on what they do to stay healthy and fit.

The secret to a sustainable healthy life lies in the eating choices we make or those we don't make every day and every time we eat. Here is how.

Many of us step into the kitchen, open the fridge, open the racks, see what we find, imagine its taste and just dash for it. There—it goes into our mouths even before we have given our mind a chance to think about what we stand to gain or lose by eating that food item.

Think—the one magic word that can make a world of change to our general sense of well-being. Thinking is the single most powerful tool that can get us from where we are to where we want to be. It is also referred to as mindfulness in the world of coaching.

Think Why

Every time you eat, think about why you are choosing to eat what you are eating and how you will benefit from it. If you have some time, look up what it offers your body (prior to your meal, preferably). It is fun sharing what you learn about foods with your friends and family and a great way of educating others too!

Think Where and When

Make a list of things you have not considered at all in your meals and be purposeful about making them available. Buy things you think you and your family should be eating and make them most accessible in the kitchen. Also, remember to find the things that you know are not good for you and stack them away (everyone is allowed a little indulgence every now and then, and how stringent you would like to be with yourself is really up to you). What is important is that you make the healthier food more accessible. Think about where you are likely to look for food and snacks, and choose those places as the spots for placing healthy food.

Say No to Junk Food

Like it or not, family and friends contribute to a lot of junk-eating habits. When we can take the kids to a healthier place to eat, why offer them junk food? It is not easy but important to learn to say no to our friends when they insist on those oily snacks or calorie-rich drinks. Try it and see how you rejoice in the feeling of being in control. Let nobody influence you on what you eat and when you eat. Plan for the in-between meal snacks. Carry salads or fruits or nuts when commuting or when you are in transit. Knowing that one has to eat healthy is not enough. One has to plan to eat healthy food too.

It will take some discipline and seemingly a lot of effort to begin with, but you will see the results, and you will love yourself for this newly formed habit. Think about it. It will make all the difference.

In essence, health and fitness, while it might seem like a personal agenda, is, really, a family imperative. Establishing a routine then, at all levels, is really important.

As a parent and a woman, you are an influential role model. If you take the steering wheel and find opportunities to pump up your activity levels every day, your kids are sure to follow suit.

Start a Fitness Regime

Fitness might be interpreted as joining a gym or simply going for walks. While starting a regime is easy, adhering to the discipline of doing something every day is the tougher part. Women share various kinds of solutions they have adopted to not lose focus on this area of concern.

Those who confessed to not being able to sustain their motivation just by themselves have successfully included their spouse or a neighbour into their regime and, in some cases, even their children.

Some indicated they did not find the idea of a gym very appealing but were thrilled about the idea of a Zumba dance. Yet others maintained that home was not a place where they could make time for exercise and chose to make some simple changes at their workplace instead. Taking a walk during breaks, scheduling walking meetings and taking the stairs as much as possible instead of using the elevator are simple ways women are choosing to use their work time productively for fitness.

Here are a few tips shared by moms who were able to accomplish their health and fitness goals:

- Identify and convert the unhealthy practices in the house to healthy ones. These range from having late dinners to snacking on junk food to eating more than necessary. Moms who did this successfully report the following key methods they adopted:

  - Throw out the junk food (most empowering and victorious).
  - Find sources of clean, healthy food. Finding healthier alternatives to the food that your family likes to eat can be an uphill task but is more like a one-time effort.

- Join a community of health lovers. Online facebook communities work great. Find local communities that hold in-person events like potlucks or cooking in groups to keep your focus and energy sustained.

- Share your wins with your friends and family. There is nothing like celebrating success, and while good health is not something we naturally tend to celebrate, it certainly is something we aspire for. Celebrations like these tend to not just motivate us to keep changing but also ignite a spark in those around us.

We are part of an ecosystem and we influence those around us with whatever we choose to do.

Reflection

- *What is your top most heath and fitness goal?*

- *What support do you need to accomplish this goal within the next three months?*

ARE YOU SAVVY ABOUT PERSONAL FINANCES?

A few years ago, I had been invited to a mentoring walk organised by a national forum for women entrepreneurs in Gurgaon. As women were introducing themselves, one woman started talking about how her husband's illness had pushed her into a situation where she was left with no choice but to learn about managing finances and running a business. She spoke about how she had always assumed that her husband would be the earning member in the family, and now, with his illness, she decided that she would need to do whatever was required as she held her family's future in her hands.

Growing up in India (and this may be true for many other countries as well), many of us learn to be dependent on the men in our families for various things, especially for financial transactions. From making investment decisions to managing household finances, we have created an ecosystem for ourselves that exempts us from being involved in financial matters. While it is helpful to divide responsibilities within a household, it is equally important for us women to ensure that we are fully aware of financial matters. We need to do whatever it takes to become capable of managing these by ourselves at any point in time without waiting for an adverse circumstance to present itself and to force us into action.

This might mean some additional effort on our part. It could mean attending a Finance 101 class to understand how to manage inflow and outflow or spending time with a wealth manager to understand the implications of various investment options. It might even mean owning a share of the household's finances and being accountable for deploying funds in a meaningful way for a secure future. Being aware of insurance policies and having easy access to the people who need to be contacted in case of an adversity and, more importantly, being able to influence investment decisions for a better future of the family are some ways in which we, as women and as custodians of our children's future, can participate in securing the financial future of our family.

It is important to think of these things before we find ourselves in a situation that is desperate, and we end up not having the time or the resources to gain these skills.

Reflection

- *Do you believe you are adequately prepared for adversity?*

- *If not, what would you need to do to be on top of your household's financial matters?*

DO YOU ACKNOWLEDGE AND DEAL WITH YOUR EMOTIONS?

Staying focused on one's agenda calls for a lot of hard work and commitment, but nothing really works if one's emotions get in the way. Most of us tend to fall prey to one or the other of the following emotions at some point in time:

- **Guilt** of not doing justice to our child, husband, household, friends, parents or our work
- **Anger** at people around us who don't seem to understand us or the situation we are dealing with, and those who constantly seem to demand more of us more than we can give
- **Regret** for the things we feel we have been unable to relish in our youth, be it material or other pleasures that seem to distract us every now and then and lead us to be caught in a moment of fleeting happiness even though we are unable to fill that void in our lives
- **Not being okay** with the way we are—thoughts like 'Maybe I am out of touch', 'I am overweight', 'I don't think I am cut out for this' etc.

Whenever we try to take a leap of faith to move forward, thoughts like these have a way of finding their way into our minds. Research has indicated that the way a woman looks has a bearing on her overall level of confidence.

What does it take to 'get okay' about yourself is the million-dollar question. For some, it could simply mean gaining more financial independence by way of earning more money while for others it might be related to a new image or a new relationship perhaps.

Our self-esteem oscillates depending on our situations. The issue with these situations is just one: we believe these situations are the means to an end. When I have this or that, I will feel better about myself. We make our happiness subject to a condition. None of these are easy conditions. By expecting ourselves to accomplish these lofty goals, we are subjecting ourselves to humungous pressure. While our goals by themselves might be excellent and in the right direction, hinging our happiness on the accomplishment of these goals is what we need to consider changing. Can we instead relish the journey we undertake?

If we were to, instead, accept ourselves and be proud of who we are and what we have accomplished despite all odds, we would, perhaps, have much happier moments. Acknowledging the power of 'this moment' is the secret to a happy and fulfilling life.

Reflection

- *What emotions do you experience the most when you are under stress?*

- *How do you plan to overcome these?*

Section 2

HOME

DOES YOUR HOUSE REFLECT YOU?

A happy home is what we all strive for—a haven after a stressful day at work, a place to relax and feel at peace.

Physical spaces in a house do have a bearing on the emotions amongst its occupants. Having spaces that are functional and purposeful can help reduce the feeling of chaos and bring about calm in the mind. A house with relaxing colors and soothing décor makes it appealing to be in.

Having one's own corner for reading or for work gives one a sense of comfort and belonging in a house.

Brian Tracy is recognised as one of the top sales training and personal success authorities in the world today. According to his research, he suggests that as much as 30% of working time today is spent looking for misplaced items. These are mostly the things that are lost because they have not been filed correctly. Sounds familiar?

Spending your valuable time looking for misplaced materials could be frustrating because no thought was given to a filing and retrieval system. Revisiting the 'homes' assigned to things of importance, be it shelves or folders on a laptop, helps in keeping information current and in removing what is not required.

The best way to organise is to place things where they are most intuitively found. It won't be like looking for the car keys all over the house just because you had left it in your jacket pocket ☺

Minimalism

If you are fond of shopping, know that an important reason to organise is to make space for the new. The space is unlikely to get created if we keep adding things and do not get rid of those that are no longer needed.A thumb rule that works is for any new thing you add, remove one. Interestingly, this applies to most things - household items, books and clothes alike.

Establish a 'Pass It On' Chain

'Removing' things can become a challenge sometimes, especially if one has no idea where to 'give' some well-maintained, expensive items. It makes sense not to throw away everything in garbage, but the important question is 'what' to pass on to 'whom'. If eventually half the things land up in the dumpster, we have only been successful in transferring our problem to someone else without adding any value to the universe. It might be worthwhile to identify orphanages around your place of stay where you could regularly donate items of use.

The other side of the chain is also having someone who is able to pass on their things to you. It is a smart way of de-cluttering and an environment-friendly way of practising minimalism.

A 'pass it on' chain would typically appear like this:

$$A \rightarrow YOU \rightarrow B$$

Limiting the things you have and keeping them where they are likely to be found with ease is a simple and smart way of saving time.

Reflection

- *How do you feel when you walk into your home?*

- *If you were to organise your home and work space better, how would things change for you?*

IS YOUR SUPPORT SYSTEM ROBUST ENOUGH?

One of the most critical parts of a happy motherhood is being able to establish a reliable support system.

It means setting up a safety net so you can take a free fall. Here is how it works.

If there are five things that you have identified as things you would like to outsource, you need to be able to find people—trustworthy human beings—who might be best placed to execute them to as close to your expectations as possible. The starting point, of course, is the identification of those key things to outsource. I know many of us struggle to begin this process, and those of us who have identified these things might want to take a look at whether these continue to be the 'only' things you might want to outsource.

How do you identify things to outsource?

Start with enlisting a set of things you least like to do. Add to this list a set of things you usually like to do but need help with often, so you can focus on other critical things.

Now think about people or sources that can help you find those who can do a good job at these things. Factor in the cost and time you need to set aside to make those options work. It is tough to outsource all things at once, so prioritising the top three might help. Would it be cooking or buying groceries or babysitting or filing your taxes or all eventually?

The key point to remember, of course, is that anyone who works on a task for you is not you. That is a different person with a different mind-set, with a different set of experiences, with a different set of skills and a different take on what is required to be done. While it is your job, and a challenging one at that, to align that person to your way of doing things, it is important that you realise that not everything can be exactly as you want it to be at all times. You would need to live with imperfection, and you would need to learn the fine art of balancing your expectations with another person's thinking capacity and capability. This would apply as much to any family members you might outsource your work to as to any domestic staff who might be best placed to help you with those 'unwanted' tasks you have enlisted.

Reflection

- *In what areas can you create a better support system?*

DO YOU NEED A VIRTUAL ASSISTANT?

We all know that post-childbirth, one of the biggest challenges that we women face is that of child care. Some of us tend to hire nannies yet live in a huge amount of guilt as we work through our day while worrying about groceries, fixing leakages and trying to keep up with our social engagements.

We grapple with what is possible and what is impossible to humanly accomplish, hoping for miracles to happen and for an hour to be longer than it is. Unable to keep up with this kind of pressure, many women tend to leave the workforce, only to find after a few years that their self-esteem and self-confidence has taken a hit and that they feel terribly unproductive managing just their home and kids.

Corporates all over the world are battling this phenomenon and are leaving no stone unturned in providing working mothers the support they need. The result is a marginal improvement in their retention rates though no earth-shattering results have been reported.

Having been through the journey of a working mother myself, I realise now that a lot of the 'stress' is really about not being able to manage the zillion of tasks that we believe must be completed. The game changer could be the 'task doer'. These tasks must be done—that's what we believe—but, guess what, *not necessarily by us.*

What do I mean? Think about it. When I was working with my coach, we listed out all the tasks I was doing in a day and found that at least 40% of those tasks could easily be done by someone else. The million-dollar question then is *by whom.* We all know how some fathers might be busy all the time, especially at the time when they are needed the most. The domestic helpers might decide to play truant, not to mention how the children may choose to be at their uncooperative best when the support system seems to be caving in.

At times like these, especially for those of us who live in nuclear families, who does one turn to? Enter a virtual assistant! Who? Exactly. A virtual assistant is like your own personal secretary or executive assistant who can do things on your behalf. What do you do when you run out of groceries? You buy them. Why not buy bandwidth instead?

Virtual assistants may not be able to do everything you want to get done in a day with the same flair as you might, but guess what, they can do an awful lot. They are available everywhere, and because they are virtual, you can find one within your budget. A virtual assistant is a person whom you hire to outsource your work to. What kind of work really depends on what you do. Say, you are in a full-time job. A virtual assistant could do online grocery shopping for you, could search for birthday gifts and send you a few options, and could even call a plumber for you when you are not around. Say, you are an entrepreneur. What are the things that bog you down? Outsource them to a virtual assistant, be it maintaining your website or following up for payments or even pulling out the latest research for your newsletters. If you are a stay-at-home mom, drowning in overwhelm, a virtual assistant might help in getting some house-related tasks off your plate while you are able to make more time for yourself. That could include lining up interviews for hiring domestic helpers or tutors for your kids or organising a party by recommending catering options within your budget.

Find it too expensive to hire a virtual assistant for yourself? Explore a share option. Many service providers offer flexible packages, and it does merit some research. If there is one way that money can buy a mom some peace of mind, this is it.

Hiring a virtual assistant can be an interesting way of improving the quality of your life even if it is just for you to take a break from all the work. You do have to pay for it, but we have already established that your time is precious.

Reflection

- *What are the top three things at work or home that you would rather have someone else do?*

Section 3

CAREER

HOW DO YOU VIEW YOUR CAREER?

Many of us spend time thinking and rethinking our careers at important junctures of our lives. A marriage, birth of a child, relocation and elder care responsibilities all tend to play a critical part in shaping our view of a career.

Women are known to scale down their ambitions post-childbirth (Source: Sylvia Ann Hewlett, *Off-Ramps and On-Ramps*). It is important to acknowledge that this is not a good or a bad thing. It is not anything to be ashamed of or be worried about. There is no right or wrong answer when it comes to making one's career choice especially post-motherhood, so let us first be okay with our choices.

A smart career perspective is that of continuity. Whatever one chooses to do, be it quitting one's job to start a business or taking a short break and getting back to a new role or even taking a break for reskilling oneself, the 'continuity' factor is important. Many women who have contributed their stories for the purpose of this book reported a lack of confidence when it came to reapplying for a job after a break, and many of those who did make it ended up quitting their jobs yet again, owing to disillusionment with the organisation or, in some cases, a mismatch between their view of a full-time job and the expectations of the organisation.

There is really no formula for continuity of one's career although, typically, a break of three to six months is good to help one rejuvenate to get back to one's ongoing career path. Longer breaks, which include some amount of reskilling or even stints at entrepreneurships, could potentially result in a substantial change of one's career trajectory.

The key to remember is that there could be circumstances in the lives of some of us that might render us 'off' our regular career path for longer than expected.

Hopefully, this is a transient period and would pass at some stage, though while it lasts, it is important to be okay with not working. The chapters that follow in this section focus on strategies on how we can be successful at whatever we choose to do.

DO YOU NEED A QUIT STRATEGY?

Celebrate endings, for they precede new beginnings.

—Jonathan-Lockwood Huie

Contrary to popular belief, quitting is not always an act of cowardice. In fact, sometimes it takes more courage to quit than it does to go on. When the quit bug stirkes, it is tough to stay rational and often, emotions tend to get the better of us. The best strategy is to wait it out, keep a check on your feelings and monitor the frequency with which you think about quitting. The question to ask is not 'when to quit' but 'what next'.

There is always that iota of doubt that might exist because it is not easy to give up something that defines you. Quitting means accepting the truth that something is amiss and believing that we can change our reality. Most of all, quitting means bracing ourselves for change and taking that leap of faith. It could mean another place, a new company, an alien role, a different set of people or anything else.

Thinking of making a shift can be overwhelming to say the least. Seeking approval of those around us may not always be the best way forward. The person who is in the midst of a situation is the person who is best placed to evaluate the pros and cons of a situation. It is important to have a winning mind-set even when quitting. Every experience teaches us something, and it is important to acknowledge the learning that has empowered us to make the decision to quit.

Here is a perspective to consider: Quitting a job, giving up one's career to take a break or pursuing other interests opens up an infinite set of possibilities.

Like everything else, there is a best practice to quitting too. One of the keys to a happy quitting experience is advance planning. Experts say that you can mitigate some of the risks by deciding what's next before you leave. In an interview for an article in *Harvard Business Review*, career planning experts Daniel Gulati, a tech entrepreneur and co-author of *Passion & Purpose: Stories from the Best and Brightest Young Business Leaders*, and Leonard Schlesinger, the president of Babson College and co-author of *Just Start: Take Action, Embrace Uncertainty, Create the Future*, agree that it's better to have at least a hunch of what you want to do, if not a full-fledged plan, before you quit.

The better planned you are for dealing with the after-life, the happier you are likely to be after you quit. In effect, consider quitting as a strategic decision and not an emotional one.

Be the queen of your destiny. You choose what to quit, when to quit and on what terms. The best way to increase your chances of happiness in the long run is simply to plan for it.

Reflection

- *What emotions does the thought of a new career stir within you?*

HOW CAN YOU BE OKAY WITH YOUR CAREER BREAKS?

While, on the one hand, corporate India is talking about witnessing a demographic dividend, on the other hand, it is grappling with the very challenging situation of women 'not wanting' to get back to work. While it is important to be doing 'something', preferably something in line with our life's calling, it is certainly okay to take some time off from work to figure out what one would like to do. Some of us tend to take a break when we believe our family needs us to. We might even want to fulfill expectations of people around us by being more available and physically present than we have been.

What happens in this 'time off' is of key significance to every working woman who has taken or is planning to take a break. The break referred to in this context is not a short-term leave of absence or a maternity leave, both of which provide for career continuity. These are, in fact, career breaks. These could last from a few months to many years and could be hugely helpful in enabling the right choices for one's life and career.

One thing with many of us is that, while we take that step forward and take the break, we may not always think of it as a smart thing to do. Let us start by getting one thing clarified: taking a break is a smart thing to do.

In marathons, in a car race, in a chess championship—in anything—a break is an opportunity to refresh, rejuvenate and restart. What we do in the break is more important than how long the break is. Research shows that most women who take a break tend to spend their time off to work around their home and focus on their neglected or compromised health.

A lot of women spend time indulging their kids, caring for their parents and catching up with their friends and loved ones. Some enjoy engaging themselves in hands-on volunteer work in their community. There are also quite a number of women who choose to get out of the rigid work formats and hunt for flexible employment options. Nowadays, there are a plethora of women centric organisations that work towards creating and enhancing flexible career options for women.

Having discussed various scenarios, it is important to remember that the thing about taking a break, is that it gives you the opportunity to fulfill many of your unstated needs and leaves you a happier person. If you plan it well, that is.

Reflection

- *What is your plan to be productively occupied when on a career break?*

- *Who can support you in creating and executing a plan that would work for you?*

IS IT TIME FOR YOU TO GET BACK TO WORK?

If you feel it is time to get back to work, consider following these simple steps:

- Start with identifying your goals for getting back to work. What do you want to do? Is it to be financially independent, is it to do work that makes a significant impact on the society, or is it to keep yourself productively occupied? Many times, we tend to miss thinking about this and might land ourselves in the wrong kind of job, only to realize that it was a mistake and then quit again.
- Next, list down your constraints. Skipping this step would only create bad blood between you and the employer. Hence, it is important to not only acknowledge your constraints of work time, leaves expected and flexibility required, but to also have an open discussion about these with your prospective employer. Is a job really a practical option for you?
- Establish your financial target. How much do you want to earn? Is money critical to you? How much can you realistically make given the constraints, skills and the experience you have?

- List down the resources you require. Do you need some money to invest in your résumé or to reskill yourself? Do you have an adequate network in your city and virtually to enable you to get the desired job? If you have decided to become an entrepreneur, how can you get plugged into networks of women entrepreneurs?
- Still confused? Get a coach. There is an abundance of coaches available nowadays who specialise in helping entrepreneurs launch their business and those who specialise in helping you identify the right career option for you. Coaching is about getting that much-needed clarity and push in the right direction. Why hire a coach? Well, why not?

Reflection

- *What is your plan to ensure you will succeed when you return to work?*

- *What can you learn from the women you know who have been successful in sustaining their career after a break?*

HOW CAN YOU MAKE WORKING FROM HOME WORK FOR YOU?

Whether you are a mompreneur or in a full-time job, working from home is the way of the future and is increasingly becoming a common practice for working moms.

Working from home saves time and cost, allows you to be more productive and keeps you away from office distractions. Moreover, being at home allows you to tend to kids, get housework done, run errands and even leave time for the odd socialising.

While it might sound like a cakewalk to some, it is definitely tougher, albeit more rewarding, than working from office.

If not planned well, working from home can result in a feeling of 'being lost' and can leave you yearning for social interaction. None of these factors are, however, worthy of stopping you from taking a shot at making this work.

Women who work from home shared the following best practices for making it a success:

- *Establish a routine* – One of the most significant and toughest aspects of working from home is creating a schedule and adhering to it. This includes the time you are done with your morning chores and start your work to any breaks you might plan during the day. A week's schedule is the ideal way to go as it allows for chunks of time to be kept aside to deal with the must-do tasks at work and at home.

- *Set ground rules* – If you are hooked on to munching on snacks or habitually get involved in every household chore or if you tend to get distracted by a doorbell or the phone ringing, set expectations with friends and family about your work time. Setting boundaries for yourself in terms of duration of breaks, TV time and time for other activities is important as well

- *Set up your support team* – If you have younger kids, having a dependable and trustworthy support system is invaluable. This includes investing in a professional caregiver or a day care even if it is for a part of the day. This is absolutely worth the effort especially if one's family support is missing.

- *Have a dedicated workspace* – Designating a space in your home is important to your productivity and your ability to focus. Have your own desk, a comfortable office chair, file cabinets, organisers, printer, a good-quality internet connection and anything else you might need to make it a functional, stress-free setting.

- *Find ways to rejuvenate* – Working in isolation can get tiresome after some time. Indulge yourself once a day with a good walk around the neighbourhood or a coffee with a colleague or anything else that works for you. The idea is to make use of the fact that you are at home and can afford any of these luxuries. Why not make the most of it while adhering to your schedule, of course?

Reflection

- *What do you need to do to ensure that you succeed at working from home?*

HOW DO OTHERS EXPERIENCE YOU?

You're never too old to set another goal or dream a new dream.

—C S Lewis

We live in a world where we are constantly being shaped by our surroundings, and everything around us plays a part in changing us into someone we never knew we could be.

As Asian women, most of us spend our lives living up to the expectations of the people around us. Like it or not, we are brought up to believe that addressing the needs of others around us is more important than living our own lives. We don't realise it, but before we know it, we have succumbed to this belief and adopted it as our own, perhaps because fighting it and wanting to live our own life takes far too much effort.

If you find yourself in this category, know that you are possibly trapped in a hideout, which is a reason (read: excuse) to stop ourselves from doing the things we truly want to do. I cannot do this because my husband or because my child or because my in-laws or because my boss—the list goes on. Interestingly, there are abstract hideouts too, like our income or our looks or—and this will sound a bit ridiculous, but it is true for some—even our skin colour. I cannot do this because, I cannot wear this because, I cannot go there because etc.

The point is that we all tend to live in these hideouts endlessly unless we are compelled by some circumstances to pull ourselves out of this inertia. The sad part is that, in some cases, the reason to break free never presents itself; and if it does, it arrives too late when our desire to live it up has receded into the valley of hopelessness.

I would argue that each of us has one or many hideouts, though the truth is that each of us is capable of recognising our hideouts and abandoning them for good. It requires courage and means facing the real world with all its opportunities and challenges. It means saying no to things that no longer work or make us unhappy and going out of our way to do that one thing that we have always wanted to do.

'People need to understand their strengths, their weaknesses, their passions, and their own story,' says Robert Steven Kaplan, a Harvard Business School dean and the author of *What You're Really Meant to Do.*

Expert on reinvention, John Mayer, a professor of psychology at the University of New Hampshire and the author of *Personal Intelligence*, says reinvention really works if we are able to find concurrence between what really matters to us and who we aspire to be. Sadly, too often, our future plans are influenced by other people's guidance or expectations. These can create pressures that can detach us from our core values.

In today's competitive world, we all realise the necessity to build a positive first impression. Whether it is a job interview, a first meeting, or a new job or role, success depends on the image we project and first impression that we create. Research shows that it takes just three seconds to form a first impression. Further, it has also been proven that people's insights are strongly swayed by the image we project.

If you are confused where to start, try hiring an image consultant. An image consultant is a person who is trained in analysing your current lifestyle and choice patterns and can provide you with some useful tips on how you can project the kind of image that you want. A good image consultant would go beyond your appearance and also get into discussions related to your communication style, which can have a telling effect on various aspects of your life.

Reflection

- *Who are the people that are important to you?*
- *How do you want these people to perceive you?*
- *What do you need to do as to create the right perception about yourself in their minds?*

WHAT CAN YOUR NETWORK DO FOR YOU?

This chapter includes excerpts from my interview with strategic networking expert, coach and speaker Paritosh Pathak, who was a guest on my radio show series 'Me in MothErhood' on the International Life Coach Radio on Blogtalkradio.

Connecting with people and building relationships is perhaps the single differentiator that we need to focus on in today's world of interconnectedness and infinite possibilities.

Many of us tend to use the words *socialising* and *networking* interchangeably. Firstly, let us understand the difference between socialising and networking. Socialising is about making the time to meet people and have fun. Networking, on the other hand, is the process of building quality and graceful relationships with people who we want to know better. The art of building lifelong relationships can do wonders for one's career and business.

Networking does not have to be a serious chore. The question is, how can you have fun while networking?

If you are one of those who dread dressing up and turning up at an event where you barely know anyone, try this technique, that we coaches call visualisation.

It is a great tool that has helped sportspersons win time and again. Here is how: Imagine that you are returning from this splendid party and have had a great time! Work your way backwards. To have a great time, what do I need to do? Look good, for sure. Go on, indulge yourself. Get creative with what you wear.

Think about how you would want to engage with people. What would you want to talk about? Has there been something on your mind you want to know more about, or is there something you are dying to tell someone? Is there someone you know who might be in the least bit interesting whom you could consider talking to? And really, this does not imply planning for a flirtation, but it could really just be a simple act of thoughtful networking. Hear more about what a couple of women whom you can connect with might be up to. Find out more about the recipes of the food you like. The point being, do whatever it takes but choose to make it a fun time for yourself.

How do you really go about building a network?

Does the idea of a 'networking event' give you the jitters? Here are some tips for you to ace any event and get the most for your network:

- Start by telling yourself that you are going to meet new people and identify those whom you would like to add to your network. When you meet the 'right' people you resonate with, make time to get to know them better. Sow the seeds and wait patiently for the relationship to grow. In networking parlance, this is referred to as farming.

- For a positive outcome, resist the desire to talk about yourself and instead focus on the person you are talking to. Try to understand the other person, their business/profession, where they come from and how they got there. By this selfless act of offering and not expecting anything in return, you will help them remember you.

- Use active listening when the other person is speaking. It not only helps you understand them better but also shows your respect and courtesy for them. It is okay to share relevant information as long as we remember that the conversation is not merely a transaction but a sincere attempt to create value.

- There is nothing wrong in being the 'closer' in a conversation. Some ways of closing a conversation are 'It was great meeting you', 'I'd love to stay in touch', and 'Can we exchange cards?'

Focus on adding value to your relationships, and you will eventually be sought after for your professional services.

In this age of social media, while building virtual networks, associated risks need to be taken into account and managed appropriately, especially by women.

It is useful to learn how to utilise social media strategically and to start building our network inside out. That would mean that we first add people whom we know to our network. We then take a brief look at people whom they know and try to connect with them. This way of reaching out to new contacts is a way of ensuring we build a 'safe' network.

Virtual networking is not a game of numbers or about how many connections or followers we have. It is about the quality of our relationships. A safe way to keep our online network relevant is to identify the people whom we do not really know and to remove them from our list.

Reflection

- *What is it that you want your network to think about you?*

- *What do you need to do to accomplish this?*

Section 4

RELATIONSHIPS WITH ADULTS

DOES YOUR SPOUSE NEED TO 'BE MANAGED'?

In urban households, where many of us work very hard to do that extra bit to get to that next milestone—a bigger house, a bigger car, more investments and more vacations—we do sometimes find that our relationship with our spouse takes a hit.

High levels of stress, lack of sleep, rationed time to talk, limited opportunities to be with each other—all these can take a toll on a relationship.

Like everything, relationships need time and effort invested in them to grow. Setting some time aside to spend together as a couple can give both partners the opportunity to unwind, rewire and relish each other's company.

Women who reported healthy and happy relationships post-childbirth reported a commonality: that of an open and ongoing communication channel with their spouse.

Some ways in which happy couples manage this are as follows:

- Going for walks or any other form of fitness like cycling or swimming provides a good opportunity to discuss the day's happenings while keeping fit.
- Planning 'dates' with the spouse during the day or a romantic evening out once in two or three weeks

is very doable provided both spouses are committed to making this work.

- Fixed routines like morning tea/evening dinner go a long way in ensuring that a certain amount of communication does happen.
- Celebrating small occasions or wins like a new house or a new car or a new job can instill the feeling of a high and create a sense of excitement.
- Working together on a plan for the future helps the couple steer the relationship forward while keeping afloat.
- Some couples take a vacation every quarter, be it a short weekend break or a long holiday to a place of common interest. Some combine trips with friends and family, though couple breaks are separate and that time is non-negotiable.
- Providing the much-needed 'space' to your spouse off and on goes a long way in keeping the relationship healthy. Be it a stag evening out with friends or a much-longed-for road trip, being able to stand by a spouse's decision to take such breaks helps in fostering trust and strengthening the relationship.

Reflection

- *What is your vision for your relationship with your spouse?*

- *What do you need to do to make this real?*

HOW IMPORTANT IS YOUR TIME WITH FAMILY AND FRIENDS?

I know, I know, too busy at work or just being at home or trying to be a supermom? We all are! Moms often have a zillion reasons why they think they can't have a social life. It is true that when you are a working mom, there are many things to manage; but too often, it is the excuses that stop us from making time for ourselves. Our days and nights are spent catering to the needs of our family, and it seems that every ounce of energy we have, goes into making sure everything is under control. The attention and care we give to our family and work is certainly important. However, it is critical to maintain our own sense of balance.

There is no stress-buster like a light moment shared with a family member or a friend. Having outlets for stress relief are extremely important. Keeping friendships intact takes more than just intent. As bizarre as it might sound, sometimes it might mean making an entry on your calendar with a reminder so it becomes a part of your schedule. Scheduling a weekly activity to reconnect with friends or your family will keep your batteries charged.

When asked about their social life, eight out of ten women cited that they had been ignoring their friends and had no 'personal' friends other than the family friends they spend time with, along with their kids.

Making new friends is not always easy when you are working, but it is certainly worth the effort. Investing time in building our social circle pays off in the form of a feeling of fulfillment from being connected with others like us. Friends are good for belly giggles, straightforward advice, sincere sympathy and, simply put, some good old fun!

With a bit of a strategy, you can make the most of the time you choose to spend with family and friends.

Reflection

- *Who are the people you need to spend more time with?*

- *What do you need to do to make this real?*

WHAT ROLE DO VACATIONS PLAY IN HELPING YOU SUSTAIN YOUR RELATIONSHIPS?

Travelling in groups is not uncommon nowadays and can mean a lot of fun for children, especially for single kids. Parents can get a breather as kids can engage with other kids and can use such opportunities to indulge in some 'adult only' activities. Homestays are a great option and preferred over hotels by many families nowadays. They provide for customised food options and usually a larger and safer play area for children.

Picking a relatively lesser-known place instead of a place that is run of the mill does have a charm of the unknown and makes for a more interesting travel.

Participating in rejuvenating retreats set in scenic surroundings can prove to be amazingly refreshing for the mind, body and soul.

Often, visualising the place that one is travelling to by doing some research, by reading about it and by connecting with some locals does build a fair bit of excitement about travelling to a new place.

'Unplanning' an itinerary is another good way of adding the zing in your travel. Keep some time unplanned in which you can decide where to go and what to do based on some impromptu information you might receive.

Dining or fishing or some such activity with the locals might seem a bit extreme to some of us women, but it is a certain way of finding out what it means to be living in the place and to soak the environment in.

Taking pictures and writing a travelogue about one's experience is a wonderful way to unwind and to immerse oneself in one's travel experience.

Reflection

- *What is your ideal frequency for vacations?*

- *How can you add 'newness' in the vactions you take?*

Section 5

RELATIONSHIP
WITH YOUR CHILD

ARE YOUR PARENTING GOALS
ALIGNED WITH YOUR SPOUSE'S?

Gone are the days when one would say 'There is no school that instills parenting' because there are such schools that exist today, and they do work. However, not all of us might be inclined to learn about parenting from someone else, and we might want to discover our own unique strengths in parenting.

The end objective of parenting, however, is for a child to be raised well. Raising a child is not an easy task by any stretch of imagination, especially when done by two different people. There will be bumps and misunderstandings along the way.

For instance, one parent might like to binge on junk food while the other could be on a health spree. One parent might believe academics are the way to success in life while the other might think academics are really quite irrelevant in the long run. Research has proven that when presented with two scenarios, human beings are more likely to pick the one that presents an easier path. The easier path that gets chosen may not necessarily be the best path for the child.

Philosophical differences that play out in the context of parenting can leave children unsure about their choices in life and might even have a long-term impact on their self-confidence.

So, what does one do? The answer is similar to what organisations resort to when they want to cascade a certain culture: alignment. Well, it might sound abit fuzzy, but think of it this way. Culture alignment, in an organisation, is meant to get employees to align their own objectives with the organisation's objectives. Similarly, parenting needs alignment too. Establishing an outcome for parenting and aligning one's own individual strengths to this outcome can produce some fabulous results.

Communication is key to any kind of alignment. If parents end up arguing about how they do things differently, it might cause confusion in the child's mind. On the other hand, when parents are able to talk about how to handle a particular situation and how to provide the child with consistent messaging, the child would be clear about what is acceptable and what is not.

In the absence of an agreement on certain aspects, dividing roles and splitting responsibilities helps. Some parents define their responsibilities such that there is clear demarcation of roles. Academics might be owned by one parent and extracurricular activities by another. In other cases, subjects in academics could be divided amongst the child's caregivers, and so could extracurricular activities.

Eventually, parenting is really about teamwork. For a couple, it is about presenting their best selves to accomplish their (hopefully) common goals and aspirations for the child.

Reflection

- *Do you and your spouse have a shared vision for your child?*

- *In what areas do you believe you and your spouse need to align your parenting?*

WHAT IS THE STATE OF YOUR COMMUNICATION WITH YOUR CHILD?

Regular open communication with our children goes a long way in helping us build a strong parent-child relationship and in boosting our children's self-confidence. Talking to our children so that they can share their experiences, ideas and worries means that we get to know them better and find it easier to deal with them when they are 'being difficult'.

Providing a window to talk about anything that is weighing on a child's mind is the role of a parent, and it could be done at any time of the day, not necessarily as soon as the child returns from school.

Conversations at mealtimes are great opportunities for a parent and child to connect. On days when that does not work, bedtime stories can be preceded by the parent asking an open-ended question to encourage reflection like 'What did you like best about today?'

Parent coaches maintain that the best way to get a child to talk and share about their day is to share about your own day with them. Eventually, children will follow suit and start talking about what happened in their day.

Here are a few tips contributed by moms we have spoken with:

- Set aside time for talking and listening to your child and for sharing your experiences.

- Be open to talking about all kinds of feelings, including anger, joy, frustration, fear and anxiety.

- Listen to your children when they want to talk. Keep your gadgets at bay as a best practice.

- Letting your children finish what they want to say shows that you care about what they have to say. When listening, try not to plunge in, cut your children off or put words in your children's mouths even when your children say something silly or wrong or are having trouble finding the right words. Children appreciate this as much as grown-ups.

- Use simple language that your children will comprehend. At times we forget that children don't 'get' everything.

- Make abundant eye-contact with your children during the conversation. Be liberal with your facial expressions too. It helps add more meaning and passion to the conversation.

Reflection

- *What opportunities are you able to leverage best to communicate with your child?*

- *What are some additional ways in which you can create new windows of communication between you and your child?*

HOW CAN YOU ADD A 'PURPOSE' TO MUNDANE CHORES?

Amidst the insanity of the gazillion tasks waiting to be done, how does one find the mental space to think about making a routine task with a child fun?

Let us take the top two that many mothers delegate or wish to outsource as they are perhaps the most testing and time-consuming.

- *Bath time* — A bath can be a special event that provides an opportunity for bonding between the parent and the child. When very young, children love to play with bath toys, especially when they are toddlers. In summers, having fun with bubbles and making a story out of bath toys create a happy bath experience. I know. Some of us who are working moms are probably thinking, 'Really? I just don't have the patience for it.' Well, it is a choice we make. If not every day, one can make an occasion out of a weekend bath. A child who appreciates music might enjoy listening to some favourite songs or learn to appreciate new ones while in the bath. Children with a scientific bent of mind might find it fun to engage in conversations about properties of water, vacuum etc. There might be yet others who are fond of fragrances, and they might appreciate nice-smelling soaps. The list is endless and limited only by our own imagination. For a chatty child, a bath can be a great opportunity to share experiences or to plan for the time that follows the bath. All this is, of course, relevant only till the child is young and still needs the parent's attention.

• *Mealtime* — For most parents today, gadgets are indispensable, even during mealtimes. Feeding a child is easy when all one has to do is stuff the food in the mouth while the child is gaping at his/her favourite cartoon on TV or the tablet or a phone. There aren't any doctors who would prescribe this method of feeding a child, yet it seems to be the easiest and a popular choice in urban households.

While sometimes it might be understandable, at most other times, it can prove detrimental to a child's eating habits, which surface much later in life. Children get habitual to eating without being conscious of what they are eating, as a result of which, they are unable to appreciate the variety of foods and are unable to make healthy choices at later stages in life. Children also sometimes engage in overeating, which can later lead to obesity and lead to further health complications.

Enough said. The good news is that meal times can be fun times too. They are great opportunities to talk about food, health and nutrition. Better still, about the day or any fun thing under the sun. Meal times are, undeniably, important bonding times almost always remembered by children even when they grow up. If you are not in the mood to indulge the child by way of a conversation, consider playing an audio story or some music. Planning a play date around meal time is not a bad idea as well as children tend to learn from other children's eating habits too (hopefully, good things!).

While these are just two of the most mundane tasks, there are so many other such things one can engage in to make them fun. Children can be involved in weekly household cleaning activities or be in charge of cleaning up their rooms. Parents can help set their children's almirahs or teach minimalism by helping children sort through their toys and accompanying them to a nearby children's shelter or an orphanage to donate toys and clothes in usable condition. Watering plants is another fun activity, especially in the summer season, when playing with water and getting wet are very welcome. Getting children to help in the kitchen by sorting vegetables or suggesting the menu for the day can even enhance their culinary interests.

Kids love playing games, and anything that has a time limit set to it can be fun and done much sooner than what one might otherwise expect. Family games planned over weekends can be fun. A walk or jog around a nearby park with your child or an hour of cycling or, better still, family days with soccer or frisbee or even good old badminton can be fun. I know of moms who joined tennis classes so they would be able to play with their kids and some who enrolled into swimming to join the fun with their child and spouse.

Reflection

- *Which parenting chores do you enjoy the least?*

- *In what ways can you think of engaging meaningfully with your child while doing the tasks you find most mundane?*

HOW CAN PLAY DATES BE AN ENRICHING EXPERIENCE FOR BOTH THE CHILD AND FOR YOU?

While good social skills are necessary to help your child lead a happier and healthier life, these skills need a fair bit of practice and training. Play dates are a great way for your children to learn to get along with kids outside school, to not only learn sharing and cooperation but also to gain confidence in their relational abilities.

In urban households, children don't just bike to each other's house uninvited. Scheduling a play date make it easy for parents to set aside time for a child to mingle with other children in a controlled environment.

Dr. Heather Wittenberg, child psychologist and mom of four, specialises in the development of babies, toddlers, pre-schoolers and parents. In her article on why play dates are important for a child, she says that a play date is an incredible experimental workshop for developing a child's social skills, and it actually boosts the child's brainpower.

For busy moms, play dates can be a welcome break, as children entertain themselves and can provide for that much-needed break for the parents. Not just that, for those of us who like to socialise and are unable to find opportunities to do so due to our hectic work schedules, play dates can provide a good opportunity to chat with other parents and discuss common parenting issues.

The kind of children one chooses to set up play dates with is, however, worth thinking about. Ideally, children might have some recommendations themselves, and hopefully we might know something about the potential play mate. While play dates with kids from school is a good idea, at times, scheduling play dates with kids from previous schools or with friends from the neighbourhood can infuse new energy into play for the child. Not just that, a varied set of playmates can make children more sociable and develop their ability to get along with a diverse set of children.

A little planning goes a long way when it comes to hosting an enjoyable play date.

A first play date is better kept short so as to allow for enough time for kids to familiarise with one another without anyone feeling overwhelmed.

Preparing your child by talking through your rules and expectations in advance is helpful. Consider establishing some ground rules like doors always stay open, no jumping on the bed, eat only at the dining table or toys be put away after playing. Most importantly, try and be around.

Reflective conversations after the play date help children play back the various events and think about what they might want to do differently the next time.

Reflection

- *In what ways can you make your child's next play date fun for both you and your child?*

HOW CAN STUDYING BECOME A 'NATURAL' PART OF YOUR CHILD'S DAY?

Establishing a schedule for a child is a topic usually met with polarised views. Some parents might believe that unplanned time devoid of a schedule is the best way for a child to explore new interests and ways of doing things. Some others tend to plan every hour of a child's day to ensure they maximise the hobby classes a child attends while building in structured play time. The in-between path is good too wherein there are some broad rules for a child to follow on weekdays e.g. TV no more than half an hour or daily one hour of studying after school irrespective of homework. Some might include educational games on the tablet or computer while the others might set aside time for handwriting practice. The right formula is yours to pick.

Every child is unique in his/her own way, be it at play or at studies. Some children are quick to pick up ambiguous concepts while some others require that extra help and reiteration in different ways. Howard Gardner has identified eight different types of intelligences that every individual has the capacity to possess. The idea of multiple intelligences is important as it allows educators to identify different strengths and development areas in each student while contradicting the idea that one's intelligence can be measured through an IQ test.

According to Gardner's theory, learning styles can vary from child to child. They could be visual/spatial, verbal/linguistic, logical/mathematical, bodily/kinesthetic, musical, interpersonal, intrapersonal or naturalist.

Identifying the learning style of your child will help you establish a study pattern easily and effectively. In many progressive schools, there is no concept of homework. As a result, children fall into the habit of playing endlessly as they get back from school. Inculcating the habit of practising concepts at home is hence extremely important.

There is really no right age to start this, but we know that kids are ready to start a regime like this as early as when they are two years old. The activity could be anything from reading books to flashing cards to building legos. Work is more like play when kids are younger and eventually changes to being more about workbooks and worksheets or reading books as they grow older.

Most children tend to get hooked on to a game or a favorite character. Being able to capitalise on this interest could sometimes hold the key to getting a child to develop interest in studies. If some children like playing Subway Surfer, perhaps they could write an essay about it. If the child is into reading, how about starting a book club to exchange books and to encourage sharing of stories with friends?

More importantly, the key is to engage the child in productive learning games whenever there is an opportunity. For children who are learning phonics, playing Scrabble helps. For those learning addition and multiplication, playing computer games like Timez Attack could help enhance their speed of calculation and give them an edge over others in the class.

Providing children with an environment that is conducive to their all-around development is imperative for their success. Designating a space for study and being around to encourage the child on an ongoing basis, are good examples of positive reinforcement.

Setting expectations with friends and family about acceptable hours of play and helping them work around the child's growing need to study is a key role many parents tend to shy away from.

What is most important, though, is for parents to use idle time to engage kids in learning games. Breakfast time, bedtime, and commute time all offer wonderful opportunities for storytelling, comprehension, word games, math games—the list is endless.

Children will study as much as they need to, provided they have adequate support and encouragement from home. If getting a child to do their homework seems like a chore to a parent, why would it not seem like a chore to the child? Children learn best from having role models. As a parent, you are the most influential role model your child has.

Reflection

- *What are the key distractions that get in the way of your child's studies?*

- *What can you do to make your children excel at their favorite subjects?*

HOW DO YOU IDENTIFY AND DEVELOP YOUR CHILD'S TALENT?

Do you remember ever thinking that your children do not go to enough hobby classes or that they need 'more exposure' to new types of hobbies or that you are unable to find ways to help them sustain interest in one kind of a hobby class? You have nothing to worry about. Most parents out there share your concern.

In any case, how does one find the right hobby class for one's child? Time, cost and distance, of course, play a big part, but the tougher part is the choice of a class. How does one choose one hobby class over another?

The one thing to bear in mind is that a child's interests can change over time. Whatever the interest might be, being able to do well at something helps a child gain an immense amount of self-confidence, which shows up in all other realms of his/her being: at home, at school and in the playground.

While attending a session by Luk Dewulf, author of *Go with Your Talent*, I discovered what I believe is a powerful way for parents to think about spotting talent and honing it in their children.

I tried to apply his thinking to the issue of parents struggling to identify their children's talent. For a child to flourish in any chosen field, the following three criteria need to be met:

- *There has to be someone who appreciates the child's efforts and accomplishments.* Think about it. If your child is a dancer or a singer, the only way the child would know he or she is talented is when people appreciate him or her for it. I know I had a tough time trying to appreciate my daughter when she started to dance on some random Bollywood song, but it took me some amount of self-talk to find a way of encouraging her dancing so as to not discourage her from dancing in the future.

a) *The environment in which a child is nurtured has to be supportive of the child's choices.* If a child is a tech geek and he is only reprimanded for touching technology equipment, the likelihood of his developing this talent would be minimised. It is easier said than done, of course. Finding a positive thing to say about the seemingly naughtiest things that a child does is not easy. If portrayed in the right manner, however, it goes a long way in developing the child's self-confidence.

- *One has to take some risks to discover a child's innate talent.* Getting a child to get off using helper wheels while learning to cycle has its risks, but the thrill that a child experiences eventually, knowing that he/she can now cycle independently, is quite worth all the effort.

Analysis of data from parents around you will show that children tend to sustain their interest and excel in classes where there is a higher parental involvement. As a parent, your role could vary from inviting the child's peers for a play date to practice what they are learning to simply being present while children practice their skills. Trying to teach children the same skill they are learning from an expert, especially if you are not an expert yourself, might be something you want to refrain from, though.

As we keep this in mind, let us play back our thoughts to when we decided to change our children's hobby class because they seemed to have lost motivation or interest.

Going back to the three ways in which talent comes to play, we might now realise that the instructor perhaps might not have been appreciative of the child's efforts or the environment might have felt a bit threatening to the child for some reason. Perhaps the child might not have felt safe to explore or experiment.

Discovering talents in children while they are young might be a matter of chance for a parent, and hence, being able to ensure that all the three factors hold good is what one might want to consider before one gives up the pursuit.

Here are a few tips shared by the moms we interviewed on the subject:

- Explore multiple activities till you find the one that the child looks forward to. It could take a while to figure out what gets your child hooked on to in a class. It might be a really good teacher or an awesome peer group or just the fact that your child is learning new things every day.

- Encourage your child to take a trial class or two before making a decision. This takes the pressure off you and off the child before making a long term commitment. Help your child to find time and adequate space for the hobby to explore it further.

- Strive for a balance of activities with studies and free playtime. Attending classes at the cost of studies or at the cost of a social life might not be the best thing for a child in the long run.

- Try to create a peer group for your child. Joining classes along with friends and family can help sustain interest and help the child learn from others as well.

- Support your children in taking responsibility for practising and honing their skills. If children lose interest, support them in making a decision and help them pick an alternate class.

Reflection

- *What hobby does your child often engage in without a reminder?*

- *What more can you do to support your children in fully exploring their potential?*

IN CONCLUSION

The key to living a happy and meaningful life is to be aware of what is important for you, at this moment, and to be committed to achieving your goals, no matter how small they might be.

A NOTE TO MY READERS AND TO FUTURE AUTHORS

The Story behind this Book

Every book has a story. There is a reason why those who write a book write it, and there is a time in their lives when they decide what they would like to write about. The why of a book is often an unanswered question that readers seldom get to know. It is a question many writers often choose to not answer, even for themselves. Here is mine.

I had known for about eight years that I wanted to write a book although it was only a year after I had quit my corporate career that I discovered my love for writing. I had no idea what I would write my book on and when. One thing was always clear, though. It had to be based on my own experiences, and it had to be for the people that I feel most empathetic towards and connected with: working women, especially working moms.

While I kept writing in different spaces – blogs, columns and my journal, it took me about a year to pull everything together: the outline, the content, the references, a publishing package and everything else.

The completion of this book, however, is largely accredited to my practice of Buddhism, a philosophy I discovered and naturally gravitated towards in 2014.

This is my first book and I will always cherish it as any parent would cherish their firstborn. I would be indebted to you if you would write to me to share what your experience of reading this book was like and how it might have provided you with a new perspective or an inspiration to move forward towards your goal.

Cheers to a life that is ours to choose!

REFERENCES

Reference Links

http://www.about.com/parenting
http://parentedge.in/
http://www.positiveparentingsolutions.com
http://www.growingafamily.com/tips/playdates.htm
http://www.drphil.com
http://www.ahaparenting.com
http://workingmoms.about.com/od/todaysworkingmoms/a/
Motherhood10.htm
http://www.empoweringparents.com
http://www.tutortime.com/parent-resource-center/
blog/2013/10/why-playdates-are-important-for-your-child/
http://www.briantracy.com/
http://saireechahal.com/
http://www.catalyst.org/
http://www.huffingtonpost.in/
http://www.realsimple.com/

Reference Books

- The Momshift – Reva Seth
- The Gift of Motherhood – Dr. Cherie Carter-Scott
- Off-Ramps and On-Ramps – Sylvia Ann Hewlett
- How to get from where you are to where you want to be – Jack Canfield

ABOUT THE AUTHOR

A **Certified Professional Coach** (CPC) from the International Coach Academy (ICA, Australia), Namrataa has coached clients across various countries including US, Europe and India. She is a **PCC** (Professional Certified Coach), accredited by one of the world's largest accreditation body for coaches, **ICF** (International Coach Federation).

A **Work-Life Integration Coach**, Namrataa founded Life Beyond Motherhood in 2012, with the vision to support women going through transitions in their career and personal lives, to help them find a balance for a happier and fulfilling life. Till date, she has facilitated over 15 conducts of her signature program– **My Life, By Design**, a life balance program for working women, covering over 300 women from middle to senior- management in various cities in India.

In her role as a **Diversity Strategy Consultant**, she engages with organizations to help create and implement their Diversity Strategy with the objective of attaining Balanced Leadership at the middle and senior levels. She has been instrumental in the success of her clients' initiatives on Diversity and Inclusion, which have received industry accolades within and outside of India.

Prior to becoming a coach, Namrataa held key leadership positions in Talent Development in leading MNCs like Accenture, Sapient Corporation, Vodafone and GE for over 14 years. Through her learning leadership roles in Namrataa was recognized for her leadership, creativity and people growth.

An avid writer, Namrataa has various blogs to her credit, ranging from learning and coaching, to her life philosophy based on choices. To know more, visit her website http://lifebeyondmotherhood.com.